Table of Contents

Understanding Anxiety Tics: Causes, Symptoms, and Management

Anxiety Tics: Signs, Triggers, and Differences with Tic Disorders

1. Introduction to Anxiety Tics

Many people with a diagnosis of mental health problems show tics. It may be hard to tell whether tics have a psychological or biological cause, as they are probably connected. When the tic is irrelevant, it should not be remembered, but it becomes confusing and less clear with respect to "anxiety tics." The following headings review the elementary aspects of anxiety tics. The definition has been defined in different ways, sometimes opposing each other. The tension in performances and situations is not uncommon: it usually arises in examinations, performances, tests, in public movements, and, in general, when there are anticipations, uncertainty, and fear of attacking others. For instance, difficulties executing spontaneous real conversation causing anxiety activated possible coprolalia, copropraxia, coperastia, or coproalgia. However, anxiety in trello vehicles is not uncommon, erupting into a neurotic block.

Anxiety tics is a broad and relevant topic within the scope of psychological and psychiatric perspectives. The present guide aims to provide professionals, as well as patients and families, with information about the main aspects of anxiety tics. For that purpose, the guide addresses several aspects regarding anxiety tics. We start by addressing its conceptualization. There are some doubts about the definition of anxiety tics, but we conduct a detailed discussion to consider its main aspects. Then, the guide discusses the main aspects of anxiety tics: its prevalence and the impact they cause in the lives of patients and families. We also discuss why it is important to understand anxiety tics for better professional action.

This post is adapted from a blog post by Duff (2015), a musician that has performed while living with anxiety tics. Clearly, there is a lot of overlap between anxiety behaviors and other movement disorders. However, it is not believed that anxiety tics and tic disorders are the same thing. Panic attacks and tics are related, but again are also different. Panic attacks can also cause or be confused with anxiety tics. This feeling of urgency to move cannot easily be resisted. If someone does resist doing the actual tic, then urges of increasing intensity tend to build up inside, and this can increase the tension in the body.

To the person experiencing an anxiety tic, it can feel like a reflex for lessening the tension and friction they feel inside their body. The muscles involved can vary but are frequently in the face, mouth, throat, or eyes. The sounds they make can be swallowed, sniffed, or hummed. These movements are the person attempting to "scratch an itch" (such as an urge, inner tension, tickle, etc.) as privately or quietly as they can. Anxiety tics look very similar to other tics and can appear on the surface to even be Tourette's, especially if they are loud or very quick. These tics can also sometimes cause injuries, due to their physical release nature.

Anxiety tics are sudden, quick movements or sounds that can resemble tics. Like tics, they often happen because of a strong urge or need for physical release. But anxiety tics are different from other tics in some important ways.

1.2. Prevalence and Impact

Anxiety tics, though understudied, occur in a larger percentage of the population than either transient or chronic tic disorders. As previously noted, anxiety tics are experienced, typically in the eye or facial muscles, by more than 1 in 10 people. Indeed, around a quarter of a college population reported experiencing anxiety tics, and a similar percentage of the general adult population of Estonia reported anxiety-based tics. The worry and distress stemming from tics tends to increase with the severity of experience. It is distressing for about 12% of people, with fewer than 1% finding the deficits in functioning significantly distressing. From the point of view of prevalence and distress, anxiety tics are somewhat comparable to other conditions with a somatosensory focus of neural symptom, such as tinnitus. Included in the diagnostic criteria for chronic tic disorders are the stipulations that "tics are perceived as voluntary, although do not have a compulsive quality" and that the individual can "Inhibit tics for limited periods". Studies show these experiences are not generally shared by those with these symptoms. Across a range of contexts and populations, we see that most people do not experience these movements as voluntary or under their control. Prevalence and distress reports differ markedly for these experiences among those engaging with them and those not. It is possible that these symptomatic experiences as diagnosed and reported are important markers for a more severe set of symptoms conceptualised as chronic tic disorders. But tangentially, the findings offer caution in generalising to the wider set of 'anxiety tic' experiences on the basis of studies primarily focusing on those in clinical settings and/or help-seeking. Given the portrayal of involuntary-movement symptoms in popular media, it is likely we receive a narrower range of feedback when seeking willing participants. Generalising the results of studies based primarily on those engaging with services is likely to overestimate the population prevalence of anxiety tics. The combination of the wider perspective and the serious impact of these movements lends significance to anxiety tics. Life largely lived in public makes any of these symptoms cause for concern and, general neglect of affective and movement symptoms, we argue, interfered with understanding their significance.

Prevalence & Impact

2. Understanding Anxiety Tics

Like most symptoms of anxiety, facial ticking is primarily neurological in nature. Anxiety can change neurotransmitter accessibility in the brain, and in some cases can actually cause the body to become hypersensitive. When you are anxious, you may remember the emotional part of the anxiety as a feeling in your chest, but neurologically your body will feel that anxiety response within the brain. Just as a flood of dopamine can result in a feeling of happiness during a pleasant situation, adrenaline can cause these movements without you trying to make them. It's important to note that not everyone with anxiety disorders will develop these tics. There are studies that have shown that the presence of tics can actually make people feel more anxious, so it may be safe to say that these are not anxiety tics, but rather tics that can be triggered by anxiety in some people. As these facial tics can also manifest in other disorders, like ADHD, Tourette's Syndrome, or obsessive-compulsive disorder, a proper diagnosis from a licensed professional is key to understanding the underlying issue. Unlike a standard anxiety tic, these illnesses cause repeated movements that can actually be physically painful in the long-term.

When it comes to anxiety, people often have a tough time comprehending what exactly it is that the individual is dealing with or what can be done to manage it. In order to fully grasp the issue, it is important for others to educate themselves on the subject. Anxiety goes much deeper than simply feeling an emotional response to a situation. It tends to have an effect on an individual on both a mental and a biological level. Anxiety disorders are becoming increasingly common, affecting 3 percent of the world population. They can cause an array of physical symptoms, from anxiety headaches and heart palpitations to facial tics that can appear out of nowhere. In some cases, these tics may actually be considered an outcome of the anxiety, and can be a tell-tale sign of an anxiety disorder.

2.1. Neurobiological Basis

Anxiety Tics The first thing to highlight about anxiety tics is the fact that they appear in any person who is stressed. Tic disorder is not necessarily present in patients with anxiety or OCD. Response tics are a relatively common occurrence in the clinical setting as well. The creation of two different categories has been suggested: primary or idiopathic-type anxiety tics, characterized by complex interactions of intrapsychic and traumatic memories, that have not emerged from any prior psychiatric or neurobiological condition; and secondary or symptomatic tics, arising in the course of, or at the conclusion of a precondition, for example, a depressive psychopathology of some sort. Although there is a wide disparity among patients with anxiety tics, some of the following observations will contribute towards the understanding and observation of those factors contributing to their manufacture. In most patients with secondary/depressive anxiety tics, the depression anxiety tics are temporary, resolving when the depression is treated.

Anxiety-related disorders have been related to alterations in activity of the gamma-aminobutyric acid (GABA)-ergic and glutamatergic neurotransmission systems and the synthesis and release of corticotropin-releasing factor, among other factors. Thus, multiple factors influence the initiation and maintenance of anxiety disorders. Physiological studies on the relationship between emotions and the expression of tics have also been published.

2.2. Psychological Factors

However, psychological factors, such as cognitions, emotional influences, and environmental triggers are suggested in the last model. The cognitive aspects that the authors suggest might be involved in the intensity or burden of anxiety or comorbid tics are about motivation and emotional expression. Here they draw from clinical observations, reported complaints in the first cross-sectional study about children (5-17 years). Deepening in this subjective aspect of anxiety tic occurrence, the factor analysis of "why do anxiety tics happen" question showed four components. The primary one was fear of missing, losing, or being disconnected from something. Subsequent factors were all about movement: findings that participants preferred the sensations of certain movements. Although the latter explains what is enjoyable about tics, it is inappropriate as a reason to guess the onset of an anxiety tic because it only answers what might make someone act on a tic if it does happen.

3.2. Psychological Factors. Anxiety tics do not occur in isolation, but arise from an inclination to experiencing distress. This shows the role of emotions. For instance, consider the strong emotions caused by an unexpected assessment. Among the emotional factors that might contribute to the inclination to develop anxiety tics are the following: (i) perceived competence; (ii) depressive and anxiety symptoms; (iii) emotional responses to the tics (i.e., perceiving them as distressing). The cognitive aspects are of importance because of the role of cognitions in the various models of tic disorders. For example, a widely recognized model of TS refers to the number of factors. Most of these relate to the neurobiological mechanisms that may be involved in the development and expression of tic disorders.

3. Signs and Symptoms of Anxiety Tics

Finally, for those who are not sure what an anxiety tic is, it's quite simple. If one feels they can't have tics unless there's a strong emotion present, be it stress, anxiety & the like, they have probably touched on anxiety tics. We call it a tic disorder if the tics have persisted for more than a year and they started when the sufferer was younger than 18 years of age. As for adults, they would have to have tics for over a year meeting the undetermined tic rule for the condition to be considered as such.

One of the hardest struggles for people with tics is knowing if a tic is a tic or not. Why does this matter? Well, if the movement or sound is introduced or exacerbated by strong emotions, particularly anxiety, then this can provide differences in how the condition should be managed. Recent research shows that the prevalence of tics in anxiety disorders is relatively high, but until recently, not much focus was placed on the potential interactions between anxiety and tics. Furthermore, for many people wanting to learn about "anxiety tics", they will be exposed to information on a well-known and beautifully unfortunate paradox: Sure, the "tic" only comes out in stressful situations, but it doesn't cause symptoms on its own, so get out of my office because what you have ain't that serious, know what I'm sayin'?

Introduction

9 min read. Commissioned by Julianna C. Zell!
Cryptocurrency wallet owners look away in worry...

3.1. Motor Tics

In general, elementary motor tics may serve to "stretch" or relax muscle groups (e.g., mouth opening is usually the opposite of mouth shutting), but it is also possible for a tic to activate the same muscles repetitively, as Ekinci has shown. Other common simple tics include hand or arm movements, shoulder or trunk jerking, and leg jerking and kicking. Motor tic events can occur in "bouts" (clustered over short intervals of time) and movements can alternate between body parts or sides of the body. Moreover, tics appear to not be randomly or senselessly distributed in time. In a naturalistic observation study, the majority of simple tics (n = 1228 of 1314, 93.6%) occurred as single, isolated movements, and the remaining 6.4% occurred in approximate rhythmic duplications.

3.1. Motor Tics. For the purpose of this article, the following part will focus specifically on motor tics. The Diagnostic and Statistical Manual for Mental Disorders (DSM-5) distinguishes between simple motor tics, which consist of sudden, recurrent, and non-rhythmic motor movements or vocalizations, and complex motor tics, which entail more complex, coordinated patterns of movements and are slower in onset. Motor tics can involve any parts of the body, and they can make use of (1) isolated muscle groups or (2) coordinated sequences of complex and sometimes purposeful movements. The most frequent motor tics involve sudden spasms of the neck (head jerks), face grimacing, blinking, lip pursing, and throat clearing.

3.2. Vocal Tics

The auditory range of anxiety tics is composed of clicks, squeaks, whistles, moans, groans, coughs, sniffs, belching, grunting, throat clearing, repetitive sniffing, stuttering, and speech block. Most adults experiencing anxiety tics come with moderate to severe degrees of discomfort, stating requests for help, treatment, and changes in education, job, or social status due to the increasing invisibility making the tics disclosed and having an impact on other people around them. Youths reverberate the fear of being diagnosed with a stigmatized disorder that can cause ejection from the peer group context. This is especially difficult for anxiety tic patients because they are overwhelmed with social insecurities in general and have severe peer-cutting deficits, hence relying almost entirely on immediate relatives and other caretakers while their private sphere seems insufficiently extended to comprise healthy possibilities for a symbiotic and fully ambivalent relationship.

Vocal tics associated with anxiety are similarly diverse to their motor counterparts in terms of type and impact on affected individuals, who come with various degrees of distress, interference, and impairment. One feature highlighted by several authors is that the vocal aspect is made up of spoken words or statements that the patient wishes not to veridically express, hence suggesting difficulties in suppressing vocal output under various stimulus conditions depending on the level of learning and associations between timing, location, and potential consequences the verbalization may bring. Awkward sensations may precede spoken verbal tics, which are generally suppressed or projected with increasing efforts in attaining secrecy and confidentiality.

Auditory Manifestations

4. Triggers of Anxiety Tics

As already mentioned, anxiety and stress are one of the biggest triggers of tics. Our body's way of releasing stress and anxiety might be the occurrence of clear yawn tics, nervous cough tics, blepharospasm, or any other automotor tics. A change in living conditions or living environment might also be a major trigger for anxiety tics. Starting a new job and dealing with new job anxiety, moving or traveling might lead to situational anxiety tics and stress tics. Those who are still not diagnosed with anxiety disorders might develop these external signs of anxiety but are still preparing to diagnose a mental disorder. Being publicly humiliated, insulted, feeling neglected, or never being encouraged are also causes of anxiety tics. Natural daily stress and accumulated stress in combination with genetic predispositions might lead to anxiety tics as well. It is always advised to identify the factor and not cover it with recommended natural products or prescribed drugs for tics but to change things that make you feel nervous and use management techniques for your skin.

Anxiety and stress are a natural part of our lives, but sometimes we might not even be aware of the development of both. Internal stress accumulates, and sometimes not addressing certain anxieties might lead to its outward expression – body tics. Anxiety tics and stress tics can come independently or co-occur with our everyday lives, especially if we develop anxiety disorder and tic disorder, among others. Some of the triggers of anxiety tics are here to help us recognize them, address them timely, and prevent more difficult mental disorders.

4.1. Stress and Anxiety

Anxiety is when a person is "uncertain and uncentered in one's mind," disoriented and drenched with feelings of uncertainty or helplessness. In this case, physical activity is increased, but without sufficient mental control, imported errors are executed instead of intentionally programmed behaviors. Across all anxiety states, hypervigilance for physiological arousal, including for heart beats and breathing, can lead to a panicked hyper-awareness that would undermine normal performance, particularly in the region of thinking and speaking. Thus, having anxiety issues could easily trigger an excess of effort and related bodily stresses, particularly when it comes to controlled and automatized actions concerning speech, thereby causing or exacerbating a tic. For tasks like speaking that already require significant and effortless influent skill, increased physical effort for any singular aspect could inadvertently highlight the lack of similarly increased mental effort.

Anxiety and its states—such as panic and stress—routinely trigger anxiety tics, and improving anxiety levels can reduce their chances of occurrence. One survey of 85 patients found that stress is by far the most common trigger, with 58% of PD sufferers noticing worrisome emotions occurring at the exact same time, and an additional 24% of patients saying regular daily stress plays a role, alongside someone saying they are also particularly vulnerable to stress related to stuttering or speaking difficulties (though it's still unclear how common this is amongst PD sufferers). Various case studies lend further support that stress often precedes the first observed tic, though this only gives us an idea of when the tics start. In one of several survey studies, the majority of parents reported their children's tics increased in frequency during anxiety-related events, while the majority of adults reported that their tics are a reliable early warning sign that stress is particularly bothersome or anxiety is rising.

4.2. Environmental Factors

Thus reducing prevent pressure on parents who find out that their child's tic may be more than just a tic, and also shortening the lengthy emotional pain of stigmatization in children who are different can also be of considerable interest. While this may be an intrusion of privacy for many families, especially in small towns where people will be able to figure out who this kid is, there feel that regardless of the invasiveness of the procedure that treatment efficiency taking place hand in hand with good faith in research should always dictate that the truth be told. There is still a deeper level of knowing within the scientific and medical community, but new information and studies tend to contradict and die out this outdated way of thinking and equip the scientist with another ammunition box to fight the old stigmatizers of generations past.

Although there are not many studies that delve into environmental factors that influence the likelihood of getting a tic, those that include them in their study serve as the base for this section. For instance, these environmental factors can take the form of having parents who argue frequently, exposure to tobacco and drugs whilst still in the womb, and owning a pet. Gathering information on environmental contribution to tics can have helpful implications for children and families. For example, using concrete findings on the causes of tics can aid parents who are unable to hear words of assurance that their still developing child will not spend his or her whole life blinking particularly hard every two minutes. They further note that many children and adults feel alone because they do not know another person who has coprolalia that they can relate to.

5. Differences Between Anxiety Tics and Tic Disorders

Most all of the definitions of these two conditions acknowledge the close similarities in the outward appearances of anxiety tics and tic disorders. In fact, some think that there are many similarities, even though the ISSPCI criteria does list some clear differences between these two conditions based on outward appearance and which ages they occur. The main difference is whether the symptoms are thought to be the result of an anxiety problem or are thought to be tics because of certain other pre-specified symptoms, features or characteristics. It is very important for your doctor to learn your individual story so that a proper diagnosis can be made, and you get treatment that fits your specific needs and problems.

Anxiety tics often look the same as tic disorders. They can involve rapid, frequent, repetitive movements and vocal sounds. These are often referred to as phonic or simple motor tics, but they can look just like those seen in tic disorders. In many people, the triggers for anxiety tics are very different than what is described for tics seen in people diagnosed with a tic disorder. It is really one's understanding of the person's diagnosed condition and the cause of their tics that determines their true diagnosis. As the field of psychiatry and the understanding of tics is an art and a science, it is important to develop a good therapeutic relationship with a physician who is understanding and willing to listen to your special story and provide treatment to help control your symptoms.

5.1. Diagnostic Criteria

The diagnostic criteria for anxiety tics define the lower limits of the frequency of the tic-like pattern and the duration until diagnosis for tic disorders. First, unlike tic disorders, the minimum frequency, pattern, and dynamics of anxiety tics were not investigated in the criteria for tic disorders. Second, while motor and/or phonic tics do not fluctuate with alterations in alertness levels and are evident before entering deep sleep according to the criteria for tic disorders, anxiety tics can disappear and reappear not only during sleep but also following wakefulness. Diagnostic criteria for anxiety tics have been proposed. Using this definition, healthcare professionals and worried people can differentiate anxiety tics from tic disorders. Then, an appropriate approach can be chosen; typically, education increases the level of confidence and reduces fear of developing complex tics and related disorders in worried people.

Anxiety tics are typically not classified separately from tic disorders in clinical practice; however, diagnostic criteria for anxiety tics have recently been proposed. Based on these criteria, anxiety tics can be differentiated from tic disorders. In this study, we aimed to investigate the diagnostic criteria for anxiety tics and discuss their relationship with tic disorders.

5.2. Treatment Approaches

The course of tics in both anxiety tics and tic disorders is often chronic or recurrent. The need for therapy depends not only on the frequency and severity of the tics but also on the degree of suffering, especially of the affected child or adolescent. For the development of an individual therapy plan, a comprehensive understanding of the nature of the disorder is particularly important in the diagnosis. Research results have suggested that anxiety tics and tic syndromes in general represent treatable disorders that can be influenced by various therapeutic approaches.

Considering possible differences between anxiety tics and tic disorders in terms of their phenomenology, course, and comorbid diseases, respective differences in the therapy concept are likely. In particular, the necessity of targeted processing of the triggering stress appears to be more essential in patients with anxiety tics than in patients with more independently occurring tics. Treatment in patients with single or multiple anxiety tics should generally be geared towards a possible underlying anxiety disorder. Anxiety can occur both with primary tics (Tourette syndrome) and as an additional disorder. There is no clinical evidence of a different therapeutic approach to primary and secondary tics.

Treatment approaches for anxiety tics

Understanding Anxiety Tics: Causes, Symptoms, and Management

1. Introduction to Anxiety Tics

Where do these tic-like movements pop up the most? Head and facial tics, for example, nose, mouth, or cheek muscle twitches. Other parts of your body can have tics too, like your arms, trunk, or legs. They may involve multiple spots in the body all at once.

Remember that tics are typically said to "come out of nowhere." And they aren't basic movements the body does to keep balanced, like shifting around in your seat. Anxiety tics are typically thought of as body or muscle tics, sometimes known as motor tics. Imagine a muscle (or several) is acting all on its own with no instructions from you. A quick, smaller jerk, like rolling your wrist, would definitely impede drawing smooth, clear lines. But not quite like the big jerk that might fling your pen off the page entirely.

Tics. "Tic" can sometimes seem like a fairly vague word. To some, it might bring up associations with speech abnormalities, like stuttering or changes in voice. For others, it might be more synonymous with tic-like or unconscious movements somewhere in the body.

Anxiety tics are both easy and not easy to pin down. When you hear "tic," you might instantly think of disorders like Tourette's syndrome. We may be less likely to connect tics with anxiety. But these spontaneous, sudden movements or sounds can still interfere with life.

1.1. Definition and Overview

Simple motor tics are brief (milliseconds to 1-2 seconds) movements that are largely meaningless, sudden in their onset, variable in their pattern, and often repetitively performed. Complex motor tics are somewhat longer and often purposeful movements that are often softer in appearance and slower in onset. Simple and complex vocal tics are commonly spontaneously loud sounds made from the nose, throat or mouth. Tics are experienced as occurring rapidly and are difficult to control. Tics may occur as an isolated episode (e.g. when under pressure) or in bursts for more than a few hours each successive day. Tics do not occur during sleep. In addition, prevalence rates of tics and/or TS are reported to be increased two to three times in people with OCD compared with the general population. There is some research to suggest that when individuals with both diagnoses experience more severe tics and detail them to have a feeling of anxiety.

To many people, tics mean movement, eye blinks or vocal sounds that are an outward sign or symptom of the neuropsychiatric disorder called Tourette syndrome (TS). In TS and other tic disorders, tics are classified as simple or complex motor or vocal and associated with sensations called premonitory urges. Anxiety or panic tics is a common phrase used to describe tics experienced in association with feeling anxious, panicky or overwhelmed. Tics can occur as part of generalized anxiety and panic disorder as well as when an individual has autism, attention deficit syndrome, and selective mutism, and when someone has different types of tic disorders including TS.

1.2. Prevalence and Common Misconceptions

Interconnectedness. Anxiety-based tics are relatively rare and are not to be conflated with Chronic Motor Tic Disorders (CMTD, which in adults we call chronic motor tics) or Tourette's. However, just as symptoms of Classic Anxiety Disorders and Classic Trauma Disorders (PTSD/PTSD-like disorders) are commonly comorbid with one another, individuals with a motor (or movement) tic diagnosis and a history of chronic anxiety/trauma likely share similar—if not the same—biological and social/cultural risk factors heavy enough to predispose them to both conditions. Further, frustration with unwanted muscle movements other than tics (dystonia-like writer's cramp), repeated, unwanted behavioral disturbances (Compulsive disorders-OCD, hair pulling-trichotillomania, skin picking-excoriation, and body-focused repetitive behaviors-BFRB's), extreme emotional reactivity or moods (e.g. bipolar disorder/depression), struggle with motor coordination and concentration (e.g. ADHD), or sensory sensitivity (e.g. sensory processing disorder), may all indicate signs of increased genetic vulnerability for tic development.

Common Misconceptions. It often surprises people to learn that stress that can bring on tics does not need to manifest as a full-blown panic attack or debilitating worry to result in a tic; consistently hearing and understanding anxiety and stress as being synonymous with these "classic" anxiety disorders can lead to missing or mislabeling lesser-seeming "bad" feelings and worries faced by individuals.

Prevalence. Anxiety-based tics are considered rare; some research suggests that fewer than 5-10% of individuals with anxiety and/or historical trauma will develop a tic, and that subpopulation will almost always have one or more known risk factors for tic development.

2. Causes of Anxiety Tics

Due to genetic predisposition: As a rule, anxiety tics are hereditary. In most cases, genetics may be the main factor in developing a tic disorder. Exposure to certain circumstances can trigger it, but it is not the cause of its occurrence. Alternatively, research by the American Journal for Human Genetics indicates that genetic history cannot have caused some cases of anxiety tic disorder. Environmental factors: Unhealthy family deficits of all kinds and (perceived non-existent) environmental support generate problems in adaptation to subjective or self-corrected physical and emotional changes to protect against traumatic attacks that would cause damage to the way of feeling and transmitting our emotions, such as the quest for an identity (which is not correct). For example, it is not the authority based on love and the personal interest of children who have learned love, but the power of authority and its law that control authority. Or that determine us as "neurotics" when gambling, social alcohol abuse, or a traumatic childhood also suggests that they are identified as such.

According to the Child Mind Institute, anxiety tics may be a more specific condition than previously believed. Individuals with the disorder tend to share certain underlying mental and social issues. Causes of anxiety tics may include psychological factors. According to the expert in Communication Sciences, Fran Navarro, they may be related to high expectations, both personal and social. They are due to the fear of failure. It is a personal experience of a negative future of guilt, anxiety, affective discomfort, or rejection that increasingly takes us away from our impulsive (choice) decision to fix us; a personal vision that excessively contrasts with our achievement expectations fixed on a high scale of preconceived social success.

What are the causes of anxiety tics?

2.1. Psychological Factors

People who have experienced tics often make comments about the way their tics are affected by their anxiety. For many people with tics already present, anxiety appears to increase the frequency and severity in tics. For others, tics appear to develop for the first time when they are experiencing a high level of anxiety. This can be quite worrying and stressful in itself and can lead to a vicious circle where the more anxious people become, the more tics they develop. It can be particularly confusing for families, parents, and friends as well as the guys going through the experience. It is not clear why some cynical behaviors may contribute to the anxiety loop. This feature can come closer to the or her tics being normal most people showing that guys showing tic response guys have normal's Diagnosis of GI for rhythm of the time.

The tics that are common can be aggravated and triggered by a number of different factors. One group of factors is psychological in nature. It has been suggested that tics may be more common in children and adults who are experiencing stress or anxiety. There is also some evidence that the anxiety may possibly increase the activity of the brain known to be involved in the expression of tics.

2.2. Genetic Predisposition

It seems that recent research is indicating that genetics can play a part in a person's susceptibility for anxiety tics. Researchers have found that tics can run in families. Not all family members may have tics, but they may have other behavioral conditions such as OCD, ADHD, or be on the autism spectrum. This can sometimes help the psychologist identify why a child is naming children with tics. It also helps the parents understand that their child is not alone. We do not know which particular genes cause tics or a tic disorder. Genes are not the only thing responsible for tics. Most people with tics do not pass tics to their children. In children and adults with sudden-onset tics following a viral illness, existing genes are thought to interact with the infection in such a way as to trigger the tics.

One of the most researched causes of tic development is genetics. Nearly half of all Tourette cases are thought to occur in people with a family history of the condition, and a strong association between genetic predisposition and tics has been shown in numerous other studies. Moreover, a significant number of tics are also believed to occur in people with family histories of OCD, ADHD, and other symptoms of what has been referred to as the tic disorders or the tic spectrum. This spectrum concept hypothesizes that Tourette syndrome, OCD, and ADD are actually different expressions of the same neurobiological condition. There are a myriad of mental health diagnoses, and sometimes tics can accompany these as well. One example of this is anxiety-induced tics, which are explored in the section ahead.

Environmental triggers of tics do not necessarily mean that they cause tics to occur. For example, Reid et al. make the point that children from those families that expressed criticism and had high expectation ratings, together with child stress, also have more overall tic severity. If a young person is less able to cope with life in general and the things that cause anxiety, then this has been found to be a significant risk factor for other difficulties. So, while being put into a stressful situation might cause a young person to tic, it might be their perception of a problem that has leaked into other areas of their life. The following section should provide detailed explanations of what needs to be included in a response to this question, which at some points require an understanding of other areas of the research.

This may be in the form of news coverage, images, or people describing experiences. One study has shown that giving details of a distressing high-stress event will make people with tics more likely to tic and increases the number of tics they make each day. Examples included an earthquake and the subsequent levels of crime, as well as higher levels of crime leading to more serious worries and the ticcing and overall anxiety the young person is feeling at the time of news exposure. Another study, interested in the effects of noise, demonstrated that "comfort noise" (such as quiet conversation) increased ticcing speed. The question "Can you tell me about the day of an important test or exam?" made these events more likely to occur in the thirty minutes following the request for information in those young people with greater problem awareness and overall feelings of anxiety.

3. Symptoms and Types of Anxiety Tics

The most common and headline type of tic disorder – as the likelihood for intervention and assistance goes – is the tics associated with Tourette's. There are verbal tics, called "vocal tics," and involuntary movements, broadly termed "motor," which allow the muscles of the body to contract and bang.

A motor tic is an uncontrollable, sudden, brief, and repeated movement or sound that has no clear purpose or cause. A person with a motor tic may hold their hand in an unusual position for a long time or blink over and over again. A motor tic is always involuntary and cannot be controlled by the person doing it. And because tics are not usually constant activities, the amount of time any individual will experience a tic, or even tics, will be modest (some tics will appear 20-30 times a minute and disappear for an hour). Sometimes a person may not tic at all during certain moments, such as when asleep or absorbed in an activity.

In ordinary forms of anxiety and stress, people may notice themselves getting fidgety or feeling the need to shake their leg. Sometimes when I'm feeling particularly tense, the muscles in my eyelid twitch uncontrollably. These are all subtle examples of somatic (physical) responses from emotional stress. But far more complex are anxiety tics, motor and vocal tics where very intense, overblown responses manifest.

As a complex system, the human body is intricately interconnected. Anxiety is part of that system and can manifest in physical ways.

3.1. Motor Tics

There are three categories where anxiety tics may be classified: simple motor tics (verifiable by direct observation), complex motor tics (requiring the performance of more complex movements verifiable by direct observation and being developed and described separately) and hyperkinetic tics (with complex motor behavior associated with impulsive sociomotor problems). Any of these motor anxiety tics can occur in an individual in isolation, and, most often, the simple anxiety tics progress to the complex ones and from there to the hyperkinetic ones, i.e., to the impulsive sociomotor problems. They are frequently associated with obsessive anxiety, a fact that contributes to greater complexity in their treatment. Anxiety tics need differential diagnosis with other motor manifestations. The causes of anxiety tics are still not completely clear. The most adhered evidence is that tics are related to genetic, autoimmune and environmental causes.

In the field of psychology, there is a general consensus that tics can be categorized in two ways: either as motor tics or as vocal tics. In casuistry, the motor tics inherent to anxiety (anxiety tics) are more frequent and are usually the main source of complaint or the reason for a visit to a health professional. Anxiety tics cause the reactions of the individuals who present them, making the school environment, professional environments or daily experiences ungratifying and frustrating. Motor anxiety tics are attacks that are characterized by sudden, repetitive, and non-rhythmic contractions of the muscles of the body and face that occur in these individuals. Rarely, the intensity of these anxiety tics carries morbidity, but their long-lasting effect may lead to obnoxious habits or problems with socialization.

If tics are complex vocal tics, there are two options to qualify their characteristics. Complex vocal tics can be either (1) modulated (categorized) or (2) unmodulated (not categorized). Complex overlapping syndrome (COS) is characterized by nonobscene complex vocal tics that are unmodulated and are usually expressed with an expression of urgency. Modulated complex vocal tic is, however, quite unusual and the best-known exhibition of this phenomenon is palilalia. This is the meaningless repetition of speech, classically uttered with dynamic inflection. When nonvolitional cognitive intrusions occur several times a day but cannot be classified as complex tics, these are categorized as cognitive tics. Compulsion syndrome, COP, and OCD all manifest vocal tics, and these tics include self-echoing, palilalia, vocalization of obsessional activity, and coprolalia.

Vocal tics are those that manifest in the voice or in other sounds emanating from the individual. Individuals with vocal tics may experience an involuntary and invariable quick sound, a long sound, or a series of quick or long sounds. Vocal tics may include different variations of hey, oh, yeah, uh-huh, uh, what, what's that, who, no, or and. Nonword vocal tics could manifest in different forms: nonword insults (e.g., fish, gooby, oy, n-a-a-a, piddle, swarthy, turd, and hell, yuck), pseudosentences (e.g., all finished, give it, go there, pick em, hey man, oh why, see you, what for, why not), or "earword" utterances that phonetically resemble words but have no semantic content

(baby, day, goo goo, gummy, lemon, no, umi-kun, and
whippy).

4. Distinguishing Anxiety Tics from Other Conditions

An anxiety tic that is briefly present, involuntarily and suppressed with great effort and perhaps emerging in seconds, is immediately suppressed when the person realizes they were focused on and observed creating the tic.

Tourette's and OCD have been recognized for a long time as a condition that creates daily repetitive movements which causally cannot be directly prevented or at least have not spread to other body areas. Because, while not directly suppressible, increases in other areas like the fingers may spread and need complex living modifications to treat.

Tourette syndrome, driven by the neurotransmitter dopamine, creates tics or repetitive movements that are difficult to suppress. Anxiety tics, driven by stress, emerge from the brain's control circuit that modulates emotions such as anxiety, anger, or sadness. It is unable to prevent these non-repetitive movements or sounds from occurring.

Management of caring for anxiety tics often involves helping the self-preoccupied or anxious individual get out of an internal pattern of fear and self-focus to engage in activities that are beneficial and helpful to others.

Anxiety tics, also referred to as psychogenic tics, are sudden, involuntary movements that accompany stress or anxiety. They are separate from Tourette syndrome tics, which are repetitive, purposeless movements and sounds with a genetic origin, and obsessive-compulsive disorder (OCD) tics. Sometimes OCD tics may look like anxiety tics, but they serve as an anxiety relief of a perceived threat and are linked to decreased distress.

Although the tics look similar, Tourettes is considered a neurological condition, while anxiety tics are a psychological issue. People who have anxiety tics often do not engage in tics if they are psychologically prepared for an event. In contrast, Tourettes makes it difficult to prepare with vocal outbursts or sudden movements. Furthermore, the symptoms of anxiety tics will disappear as soon as the anxiety is managed or the overwhelming feeling subsides, and are not affected by external stimuli. On the other hand, for a person with Tourettes, the tics are not controlled by the individual and will tic no matter the emotional state. It is important for healthcare professionals to ask questions and note the differences between these conditions in order to prevent misdiagnosis. Misdiagnosis could result in prescribing inappropriate medication.

Anxiety tics are different from Tourette syndrome. Tourettes, a childhood condition, causes a person to make repeated involuntary movements and sounds called tics. Motor tics can include repetitive eye blinking, facial grimacing, head movements, shoulder shrugs or jerks, and heavy swinging of the arms. Vocal tics, or sounds, may include sniffling, grunting, throat clearing, yelling, or high-pitched squeals. Tics can also be more complex and longer, involving moves such as squatting, hopping, skipping, jumping or twirling in circles. Voices can become involved, resulting in the use of curse words that may be socially inappropriate. People with Tourette consistently show symptoms of two different types of tics over the course of several years. It involves one or more motor tics or vocal tics that occur at some time during the illness, although not necessarily at the same time. Anxiety tics, however, are a physical symptom of anxiety and often only include motor tics such as biting nails, whiting the eyes, twisting the hair, thumb sucking or skin picking. These tics can occur at any point in life and do not have to meet the regular time frames of tic disorders. They are a voluntary action.

Additionally, there may be some overlap between people who engage in repetitive tics for explicit obsessive-compulsive disorder reasons. While this results in physical tics seeming behaviorally similar to habits performed by those with obsessive-compulsive disorder, the natural tendency to overthink in times of strong anxiety does not automatically mean that all repetitive physical tics are purposes to stave off self-doubt, for example. It can, however, mean that some techniques that work effectively for obsessive-compulsive disorder can be beneficial in treating and managing certain sequential tics as well.

Though the term might lead to some confusion, anxiety tics are not to be confused with the similarly caused anxiety disorder known as obsessive-compulsive disorder, or OCD. Those diagnosed with anxiety tics are not necessarily suffering from obsessive-compulsive disorder. Although anxiety tics and symptoms of obsessive-compulsive disorder are indeed related in that they are both caused or exacerbated by anxiety, tics represent a physical movement of the body, whereas that is not necessarily the case for everyone with obsessive-compulsive disorder. Though someone with obsessive-compulsive disorder may engage in actions because of anxiety, they may not have a physical compulsion in the same way that someone else with anxiety tics might. As such, the types of cognitive-behavioral therapy techniques employed might differ between someone with ongoing anxiety and someone with conversely reduced anxiety but still experiencing these symptoms primarily as an effect of the tic generation.

5. Impact of Anxiety Tics on Daily Life

Very severe, frequent or intense tics can lead to chronic pain or injury (for example, falls caused by motor tics). Tics can also get in the way of conversations and, in severe cases, make it difficult to communicate. Verbal tics can also make it more difficult for others to understand you, which can lead to frustration. Tics can also be personally distressing. Some people with tics describe a sensation similar to "tingling" before the tics occur. For some, this sensation may occur frequently; for others, less often. Knowing that a tic is about to occur can cause a feeling of anxiety. It may be that the tic cannot occur in a particular situation, which can lead to an increase in anxiety. Whether you work, dedicate yourself to studies, or enjoy artistic activities, tics can be frustrating. You may have difficulty staying focused or taking on new challenges. Even day-to-day tasks can be overwhelming and distressing.

Anxiety tics affect various aspects of an individual's life, including both short-term stress and long-term complications. Anxiety tics can lead to social life impacts, such as avoiding going out or spending time with friends. Being in social situations can cause people to feel more anxious and create a cycle of avoidance, worsening anxiety with time. Anxiety tics can affect emotional states. For example, there can be an increased sense of frustration, lower self-esteem, and difficulty feeling good. Regardless of academic or job performance, always relying on corrections and taking additional time can also reduce self-esteem. There can be occupational impacts, including an increased difficulty working or taking tests.

5.1. Social and Emotional Effects

Given that la belle indifférence (a lack of concern about physical symptoms) is a relatively common characteristic of a conversion disorder patient, the fact that many children and adults with anxiety tics express upset around these prompted us to acknowledge the emotional toll of these phenomena. This decision also draws attention to the social isolation that children and adults with other different presentations of tics can frequently experience in day to day life. In light of this, the pediatrician Müller must tend to both physical and emotional needs of his patients. Trudy's revealing story may open the door to receiving an empathetic and understanding response, particularly in light of her own self-critique of the 'ciphers' and 'wrigglings' that transpire as she tries to reconcile her strong stated emotions with the impactful, and her attacks on such meanings. In doing so, Trudy may tie interviewers up within the very hermeneutics she seeks to escape.

As anxiety tics are not so well understood or even mistakenly identified as voluntary behavior, these can considerably shape public and social attitudes and perception. Ultimately, this can make many everyday interactions a challenging experience for the individual. The individual's emotional wellbeing is also of importance here. As highlighted in the case of Trudy, people with anxiety tics can feel self-conscious and embarrassed about how others might perceive and evaluate them. Although Trudy does additionally express that she believes people's attitudes and anxiety about her anxiety tics are largely unimportant, the focus of her statement highlights the extra cognitive load and stresses that occur when struggling to manage how others might feel.

5.2. Academic and Occupational Impacts

Research in this field has shown the following findings: previous family history of anxiety tics (ca. 23%); tendency to worry and sustained stress (ca. 13%); poorly adapted, pessimistic thought pattern (ca. 10.5%); health beliefs of the "three poor" type (ca. 9%); prior traumatic accidents, threats, or surgical experiences (ca. 7.3%); major life events and loneliness (ca. 7%); and changes in the living environment, such as resettlement, difficulty in adapting to the new environment, long-term cultural conflict, empty nest syndrome or frustration (ca. 4.5%). The community-based study of 150 patients with anxiety tic disorder showed a particularly high school failure rate, with 85% having been suspended from school, 53% even having had suicidal ideation, 30% having failed once or twice a year, and 35% losing confidence in life after the onset of the disease. Thirty-six patients in the workplace were exhausted as a result of their unsustainable professional layer. Only 18 patients currently have relatively high academic qualifications and can engage themselves in their dream jobs of the disease biology educator, while the remaining patients have been unable to engage in other professions due to the disease.

The majority of previous literature focused on the prevalence, etiology, and medical treatment of anxiety tics. As a result, few studies addressed the effects of anxiety tics on human quality of life. In particular, a noticeable increase in anxiety tics corresponded with the beginning of the academic and occupational activities that dominate most of the day. In many schools and occupations, suffering from anxiety tics means being depressed, having trouble concentrating, and losing self-confidence. The symptoms of anxiety tics also result in the denial of many life opportunities, such as playing musical instruments, sports, arts, theatres, choirs, and interacting with pets. Emotional factors also play an important role in this underprivileged group: loss of friends, loneliness, narrow social environment, and the behavior pattern of "no friends at work, at home, no one" are significant. After a complete medical and psychiatric observation, it has been ascertained that around 10.19% of the patients referred to clinics/wards for the first time are suffering from anxiety tics.

6. Diagnosis of Anxiety Tics

The disorder that can present with anxiety tics includes other neurodevelopmental and mental disorders, such as other tic disorders (in case of more complex motor tics, e.g., due to a comorbid Tourette's syndrome), movement disorders secondary to neuroleptic treatments, other movement disorders (e.g., choreoathetoid cerebral palsy), stereotypic movement disorder, other specified tic disorders (could present as Tourette syndrome with late onset), functional movement disorders, and tics secondary to substance abuse/withdrawal. Anxiety symptoms, even though indistinguishable from other anxiety disorders, generally have a relationship with the tic symptoms. Since tics are mostly conscious, they are generally involuntary rather than purely autoimmune or involuntary, but this should be assessed on a clinical case-by-case basis. Comorbid obsessive-compulsive and related disorders, especially the separation of OCD, should be based on the nature of the preoccupations and/or their outcome behaviors rather than only the presence of obsessions.

Considering the diagnostic workup, the psychiatric assessment should include an evaluation of the tics, taking into account their phenomenology (vide infra). Furthermore, neurodevelopmental and mental comorbidity in psychiatric morbidity, symptom severity, antecedent course, and psychosocial and familial factors contribute to a global clinical assessment in anxiety tics. With regard to etiologic psychiatric diagnostics, the evaluation of risk factors and/or protective factors for the outcomes, as well as potential disorders that could have already been present, plays a central role.

Physical medical consideration is a vital portion of an evaluative procedure of persistent tics in anxious patients given that ALS is already experiencing both physical and cognitive discomfort, as well as emotional assessments for the assessment of psychological discomfort. Additionally, BCs can yield critical details that many customers are unable to communicate using words. Yet doctors of physical pain perform clinical evaluation by merely excluding both the presence of a bodily ailment and any involuntary, rather neurologically motivated, injury. Similarly, requests for regiments and IPR/SIH must differentiate between PTSD related to a health problem and hypochondria.

When a person demonstrates anxiety tics, it is crucial to seek an evaluative inventory and to have a medical check-up. Main assessment tools such as pre-selected and open-ended interviews, pending on the mode of the interview, ranging from a patient-initiated to a professional-initiated evaluation, are presented. A clinical interview yields systematic data on the patient's past and present emotional, physical and cognitive symptomatology, the course of the tics and the patients' viewpoints, findings, and worries about the tic. The questions of an evaluative interview are fundamentally dissimilar because fear or avoidance of hastening or restricting the appearance of a tic may amplify tic complaints, often with incredibly scarce psychiatric records. A review of impairments provides us with more determinative and mechanistic information in order to fully realize the tools applied by clients at large as they mitigate tics.

6.2. Differential Diagnosis

Although anxiety and tension, unlike dystonia, can cause an increase in tic appearance, other factors that provoke tics such as stress, anxiety, fatigue, and anger may not always be present. If other tic-provoking factors exist, the diagnosis should be questioned. If movements are completely coordinated with a goal, evaluated using videotape analysis and clinical evaluation, a movement disorder or an associated movement, not a tic, should be considered. Some children with anxiety tics may suppress tics, resulting in a build-up and a rebound increase in tics (inside-out tics). These should not be diagnosed as complex tics mimicking inside-out tics. Children with tension or anxiety of developing tics may behaviorally attempt to dilute the tics of others and challenge, distract, or draw attention to the tic, but these should not be diagnosed as complex tics. If resistance does not lead to the suppression of tics, then the diagnosis of a behavioral tic can be questioned. In some resistant cases, a minor tranquilizer would enable the tic to be suppressed, leading to a clear diagnosis of a behavioral tic. Tics masquerading as craziness or psychosis places the diagnosis in the differential of tourettism and OCD because there may be complexes of symptoms so bizarre that they do not correspond to either other known disorders.

Differentiating tic disorders related to anxiety and obsessive-compulsive symptoms (anxiety tics) from fully developed tic disorders, other movement disorders, and seizures with tics typically arises through clinical presentation. Tic disorders related to anxiety and/or obsessive-compulsive symptoms (anxiety tics) should not be differentiated solely on the appearance of tics. A diagnosis of anxiety-related/reasonative tics is proposed if the tics, premonitory urge, functional character of tics (suppression, reduction with distraction, change in location, etc.), comorbid anxiety and/or obsessive-compulsive symptoms, an association between waxing and waning of symptoms and anxieties/obsessions, or reduction in tic symptoms with anxiolytics such as selective-serotonin reuptake inhibitors (SSRIs) occurs. This proposal is based on the long-standing existence of the tic disorder, high response to OCD treatments, and alleviation of tics by SSRIs. The presence of a positive family history for OCDs, tics, anxiety, and mood problems is also a known factor that can be investigated to support the clinical diagnosis of tic disorders related to anxieties/obsessions (anxiety tics). It may not always be easy to establish the diagnosis, especially when differentiating from dystonia and stereotypies.

7. Treatment and Management Strategies

- Breathing and relaxation - Cognitive-behavioral therapy and acceptance therapy.

Medication There are a number of medications that may be prescribed by healthcare providers to help manage anxiety and the use of tics as a way of coping. Tics may be worsened by anxiety and can be made more difficult to overcome because of this. If anxiety tics are a significant problem for you, it is likely that medication to manage anxiety will also be considered. You may have to try a few before you and your healthcare provider find one that works well for you. Sometimes tics can become worse when you start new medications for anxiety, but this period of reaction should be discussed with your doctor. Make sure you understand possible side effects, and tell your healthcare provider about any side effects you experience. It is important to monitor your levels of anxiety, and if tics are not responding to anything, to get help to get your coping strategies under control. The following therapies can help with understanding and managing any anxiety related to your tics:

Therapy Cognitive-behavioral therapy for tics (CBT) is designed to help reduce the impact of tics on an individual's life, identify and tackle the situations and beliefs that maintain the problem, and tackle anxiety and depression, which can make the tics worse. It focuses on stress management and developing a relaxed lifestyle, correcting thinking errors and increasing the ability to reduce worry and stress. The NICE guidelines recommend this approach to the management of chronic tics in people aged 5 and older. Usually, such therapy would last approximately 10 sessions at first, although it can be offered in different formats for different individuals.

There are a number of options for treatment and management of anxiety tics, including different types of therapies and medications. People usually respond best to a combination of treatments. Keep in mind that anxiety tics are difficult to manage for both the individual who has tics and the professionals involved in their care. Everyone's experience is individual, but this page is written for individuals and their healthcare providers.

In older children and adults, service providers often ask their clients to maintain a diary that logs their physical and emotional reactions, which will help to develop their own individualized hierarchy-response prevention plan. This diary keeps a record of when and where the tic occurred, the circumstances surrounding the tic that made it better or worse, the strength or severity of the tic (i.e., mild, moderate, severe), the urge or feeling that they had immediately preceding the tic, the type and duration of the tic, and the perception of others to the tic. Some diaries have worksheets that are combined with the entries to track responses that are used during each session.

Anxiety tics, including those caused by generalized anxiety and other anxiety disorders, may not completely cease through appropriate medical interventions. In such cases, learning to cope with anxiety is a major component of controlling tics. Behavioral approaches are the most common type of nonmedical treatment available. While different theories support these treatments, the most widely studied, with the strongest evidence base, is cognitive behavioral therapy (CBT). CBT addresses the connection between thoughts, feelings, and behaviors and aims to help a person identify, challenge, and change maladaptive thoughts and behaviors to help them cope with and reduce physical and psychological anxiety. CBT, specifically exposure and response prevention, is routinely recommended by all clinical practice guidelines to manage severe tic disorders, such as Tourette syndrome, unless there is an active reason it should not be used. Exposure can occur interoceptively (focusing on the symptoms of anxiety such as heart rate and muscle tension) and exteroceptively (focusing on confronting fears in real-life situations). The goal is to decrease the physical, mental, and emotional feelings of anxiety that accompany the triggers causing the tic. Between sessions, people are asked to practice what they learned from their session.

7.2. Medication Options

In general, it can take some time and working closely with your doctor to find the right medication or combination of medications to help manage anxiety tics. Not every medication will work for everyone. Because many anxiety tics can worsen with emotions and stress, learning healthy ways to cope with and process emotions is one of the most effective ways to reduce anxiety tics. Cognitive-behavioral therapy has been found to be very helpful for many sufferers of anxiety disorders. There are also some helpful medications for anxiety. It's important for patients to work closely with a mental health provider who can accurately diagnose the anxiety disorder, discuss the risks and benefits of medication options, and monitor progress to ensure the best care possible.

Medical warning: All antipsychotic medications come with warnings for the potential risk of developing movement disorders, known as tardive dyskinesia. This risk is rare, but it is important for patients and family members to know what to watch for and to report any new or unusual movements or tics to the prescriber.

Antipsychotic medications: Some doctors find benefit in using certain antipsychotic medications to treat anxiety tics, though this is unusual. This may be a good option for some children and teens who have anxiety tics and related conditions, including autism, ADHD, or obsessive-compulsive disorder.

Blood pressure medications: Because anxiety tics and twitches are often driven by the "fight or flight" response, blood pressure medications can be helpful in reducing anxiety tics. Some blood pressure meds, such as clonidine (Catapres), can reduce symptoms quickly.

8. Lifestyle Modifications and Coping Techniques

People of all ages report that specific dietary or nutritional supplements influence tics. Some people note that increasing their magnesium intake either through magnesium-containing food sources or supplements helps them manage their tics. Other people report feeling better and reduced tics when they reduce their sugar or glucose intake, eliminate caffeine from their diet, or consume omega-3 fatty acids (fish oil). Keep in mind that there may be a connection between the level of comfort and improved individual tics, but there is no scientific evidence that a specific diet helps to reduce the frequency of tics. Given the lack of widespread or reliable techniques for treating tic, and the lack of information about the exact efficacy of the above stress reduction techniques, it is necessary to study the long-term impact of lifestyle stress reduction on tics and tic irritability and chronicity. Anxiety at tic has been associated with attention deficit hyperactivity disorder, and therefore more research on self-sufficiency in tic/ADHD populations may be required, as this method brings added value to young people with tic and ADHD.

Along with medication, encourage your child to make stress reduction a large part of their treatment plan. These lifestyle modifications can also be applied to children who are sensitive to certain activities and reduce the amount of tics they have. Usually, anxiety tics increase in environments that are particularly stressful. Stress management helps patients reduce episodes of tics and recurrences. Mindfulness and relaxation practices, such as diaphragmatic breathing, exercise, and yoga, can reduce anxiety associated with tic and help maintain or improve sleep, overall forcing, attention, and mood. Medication and psychotherapy such as cognitive behavioral therapy (CBT), cognitive-behavioral intervention for tics (CBIT), anxiety reduction training, and targeted psychodynamic care are the main treatments for anxiety and tics with lots of scientific evidence. However, the importance of other strategies for managing tics, feelings, and anxiety, which are part of living with childhood tics, has been discussed, such as training in managing signs and symptoms, information and education.

At the same time, it is also very important to note that stress can be a primary factor that exacerbates anxiety tics and makes tic ticcing worse or more severe. Therefore, we believe stress management techniques can be beneficial for those who'd like to try them out as one of the first ways to try and help themselves either reduce the amount of tic ticcing they do, bring tics under more control, or to reduce the severity of tic symptoms.

One of the most important elements in effectively coping with anxiety ticcing and learning to manage it is stress reduction techniques. Those with anxiety tics can learn stress management techniques that work best for them, or disregard those that offer no positive impacts. There are numerous different techniques that people have used to manage their stress, and for that matter, to help reduce their anxiety tics. It is important to remember, however, that while some of these techniques will prove more effective than others, none of the techniques listed below will cure ANS or anxiety tics. In fact, as of now, there is nothing that can cure or eliminate the symptoms of either condition. Furthermore, while it may be possible that some techniques might stop or prevent anxiety tics, it is also possible that no technique will have a single shred of impact.

There are stress management techniques to help reduce the impact of anxiety tics.

8.2. Mindfulness and Relaxation Techniques

How the Techniques Work: These self-soothing techniques essentially work by calming down the mind and the body, giving the mind something else to focus on other than worry or stress. Essentially, if you concentrate on the present moment, there's no room for worrying about what comes next. In essence, it combats a racing mind or an anxious conscience. These are best used around or with help from some other, more traditional, therapeutic treatment. They should not be used in place of other therapies. If you are experiencing a tic, remember that you should work on being as calm as possible. Meditation, mindfulness, and relaxation can all help. Keep in mind that it might take a while to find something that works for you, and what works for one person may not work for another.

Mindfulness and relaxation techniques have their own plan of attack when combating the anxiety tic. Unlike the exalting in the midst of chaos approach of the previous section, in this section we seek to create an anxiety-free environment externally in the hopes this will calm nervous tics. It kind of makes sense. If you don't have the stress, there will be nothing to trigger the tic. These are really just some ideas as you try to be aware of yourself and massage your mind and spirit into submission. They don't necessarily belong under the rubric of types of anxiety therapy, but the next best place seemed to be a home here.

9. Support Systems for Individuals with Anxiety Tics

A healthy body and mind need an environment conducive to their well-being, wherein one can secure fulfillment and happiness, realize one's own potential, and live life to the fullest. This inevitably involves love, care, and devotion from family, friends, and significant others. If the anxiety tic becomes more obvious and disruptive, it may become an issue for the immediate family. It is important for these people to know that every individual has a limit to control illusionary diseases, such as anxiety tics, and they require a lot of support. The most significant aspect of a supportive environment is helping those with such behaviors to collaborate together and improve the situation both at home and at school.

Individuals with anxiety tics require supportive systems to manage their symptoms effectively. The United Nations, along with various religious organizations, help create coping mechanisms for affected individuals through awareness and training programs. Presently, parents and family support individuals with anxiety tics by providing emotional support and understanding. Additionally, connecting with others in the same boat can bring beneficial effects to individuals with anxiety tics. That is why peer support groups can be helpful for individuals with the disorder. The group can discuss problems informally and set up social activities.

9.1. Family Support

Family members not only play a crucial role in anxiety control, but living with family also boosts the confidence of the individuals in dealing with their anxiety and living with others. Also, while sharing with family members, they tend to get distracted from stress and indulge in their favorite activities. Research shows that how family members support anxiety patients affects them a lot. There is strong evidence that family-provided help and support can improve the condition of an anxiety patient.

Through thick and thin, families are always there when we need them. Anxiety, whether a reason for tics or not, family plays a crucial role. Around 70% of individuals report that their family relatives are aware of their tics. In another 40%, family members also experience their close individuals' tics. The odds of continuing the habits and behaviors tend to increase if any local relatives are aware of them. Therefore, it is important for one's relatives to have enough knowledge about their tics. This can help build a sense of self-awareness and familial participation. Those individuals' relatives who are aware of their tics tend to know better about the results of their behavioral habits and habits. They are also more aware of the consequences of their behavior and help them to live in harmony with others. Along with all that, they also help them learn to be aware of others when going through tough days.

In addition to chat room support and other resources, the following support groups are available for help with anxiety tics. However, it is best to check with your local organizations: BFRB.org, also known as the International Centre for Excellence in Body Focused Repetitive Behaviours, has a collection of resources on this website for finding trained professionals near you. It also offers an online story-sharing project called #ISeeYouWithBFRBs. The TLC Foundation of BFRBs is another great resource. It has an 'Are Support Groups for Me?' page and a link to the 'Find Help' section, which lists local support groups, online and virtual support, online events, and webinars. The Association for Behavioural and Cognitive Therapies also lists the following evidence-supported support groups throughout the U.S. on its website.

Many individuals with anxiety tics find that meeting others who have similar experiences with picking is one of the most encouraging things they can do. We know from personal experiences that others with tics can often understand the problems we are facing better than those who do not pick. Many who obtain professional or medical help for their anxiety tics report feeling let down or misunderstood by the professionals and found more relief from speaking with others who have the same compulsion. Knowing that there are others who can offer this kind of support when you are anxious can also give you more confidence to lower the amount of skin picking you do. Recently, some people who have tics have started reaching out to others through the Internet by creating chat rooms, support groups and services so they can offer each other understanding and advice. Some of these tics are also very good in referring to professional help if it is needed.

10. Research and Future Directions

For some cases of anxiety-related tics precipitated temporarily by high levels of anxiety experienced by a person whose underlying worry or fear is of losing control or engaging in uncontrolled movement (rather than by a comorbid tic disorder), can be normalized with exposure therapy or habit reversal, depending on the treatment-relevant factors. Exposure may be contraindicated for youth with high levels of social anxiety or other fears and should only be used in such cases with additional psychosocial support for the youth and consultation with or assistance from an anxiety treatment specialist. Published findings examining the empirical support for psychosocial treatment of anxiety-related or secondary tics are scant, although such research is ongoing. Also, most anxiety-related tics are mild. So, pharmacotherapy is not usually necessary for the specific management of most tic suppressors. Some studies have shown that antianxiety medications and selective-serotonin reuptake inhibitors (SSRIs) can improve some secondary tics. More focused anxiolytic medications can improve anxiety and in some cases anxiety-related tics, but there are no medications specifically indicated to decrease just anxiety-related tics either generally or as a class, such as those whose presence might be targetable by an experientially based cognitive behavioral treatment. There is also evidence that tourettic persons with moderate to severe anxiety have more severe tics that are more difficult to control. Research is ongoing.

Examination of anxiety-related and non-clinical tics may help explain the wide range of tic expression and course seen in TS and may also clarify clinical presentations seen in patients with comorbid tics and anxiety-based symptoms within major chronic motor tic disorders, such as provisional tic disorder and chronic motor tic disorder. It may be that presentation and course are influenced more by the presence or absence of underlying tic diathesis than by anxiety level alone. With this understanding in mind, future empirical research on anxiety tics in general should focus on testing moderational or mediational effects of underlying tic diathesis on the relationship between anxiety and tics. Furthermore, such a conceptual model would better help guide treatment.

Another condition that can be managed with the right response. The launch of this research has proven to confirm what we've known all along; much is unknown about anxiety tics, except that they are a reflexive response to intense emotions. Although other reviews from researchers claim to have information about the "cause," it is still thought of as a medically "medically unexplained" condition. There are some factors that are consistent for many sufferers, such as the increased heart rate as mentioned previously in this report, but there are often underlying conditions and/or other comorbidities that make systems a unique experience for an individual. What does this tell us? It's an unfortunate truth, but not much. Depending on each individual scenario, it may or may not be problematic; treatment and reaction depends entirely on the individual and the experience.

When it comes to anxiety tics, there may not be a great deal of information available, but studies and research continue to be carried out to further our understanding. What has been discovered in recent studies is as follows: An analysis of worldwide research between June 3, 2020 and November 1, 2021 that was released in Scientific Reports has given us a bit more insight about tics in general. Known as exploratory tic behavior, the act of the arms and hands moving to a new position rather frequently, is more likely when the subject is fatigued, while a subconscious change in posture known as tachypsyopagis (meaning rapid scrambling) is also correlated with the act of tic behavior.

Section 10.1. Current Studies and Findings

Spicher and Janki reported a 15-year-old male child of Hispanic origin with intellectual disabilities assigned etiologic cause between genetic and acquired (following an episode of febrile seizure and other minor seizures), compensated hydrocephalus, without a perinatal background or services, who presented himself with classic FOS (facial onset seizure), with manifestations that clearly denoted motor and sensory phenomenon of partial versive seizures (head to the left) with preserved awareness. When the child was exposed to natural sounds and light, the phenomenon completely disappeared including the signs of anxiety. The association of anxiety in FOS is not known phenomenon. The principal treatment for these events usually involves the use of antiseizure medication. By using these findings, one would favor the ratification that the case represented FOS. It is also possible that the child may have a phenomenology that could also be considered anxiety tics or anxiety nonepileptic events due to psychopathological considerations. For the case at hand, the seizure disorder aspect is not the prominent concern as there are rare cases of observing self-induced seizures and a permanent cure following puberty without AED. Also, the boy is currently asymptomatic with the finding of mild and regular epilepsy even after having stopped the treatment of recruitment methods.

10.2.2. Natural Sound in the Clinic as Potential Therapy for FOS

Vergne and Luis Almeida reported an 18-year-old woman affected by Down syndrome with severe PIMs for the previous 5 years, everyday, regardless of the circumstances. A diagnosis of anxiety tics was retained. Alprazolam (1 mg/day) did not lead to any improvements on the follow-up of the patient. During a visit to the dental department for dental care, she received general anesthesia for intravenous sedation according to a protocol comprising the injection of propofol (2 mg/kg body weight, bolus) and fentanyl (2 g/kg). Unexpectedly, a significant, immediate and repeatable improvement in maintenance of the complete disappearance of tic-like movements in the arms, allowing dental care to be performed easily, was observed. It was decided to re-induce general anesthesia for both the same purpose as during the prior episode, and also to verify the robustness of the phenomenon during the entire procedure. Retesting before dental care was performed without anesthesia and tic-like movements were easily induced. Repetition of dental care with propofol-fentanyl anesthesia resulted in re-induction of immediate, complete and lasting disappearance of tic-like movements in the arms.

10.2.1. Anesthesia for the Prevention of Repetitive Tic-like Movements